LET'S TALK ABOUT

MENTAL HEALTH

Brenda A Thigpen, RN

authorHOUSE®

AuthorHouse™
1663 Liberty Drive
Bloomington, IN 47403
www.authorhouse.com
Phone: 833-262-8899

Published by AuthorHouse 12/14/2023

ISBN: 978-1-6655-1179-7 (sc)
ISBN: 978-1-6655-1180-3 (hc)
ISBN: 978-1-6655-1178-0 (e)

Library of Congress Control Number: 2020925671

Print information available on the last page.

Author's Intro

My name is Brenda Thigpen, born Brenda

Haywood to my parents, Yvonne

Bristo and Claude Haywood

Dedication

I would like to dedicate my writing

to my grandparents:

Maternal: Edna and Phillip Bristo

Paternal: Lenora and Jonathan Haywood

Special reference to Dr, Hyacinth

Martin, my friend and mentor.

The Purpose

The purpose of this book is to assist parents, other family members, and perspective clients in making the decision to seek help should they experience signs and symptoms of possible mental health issues.

Goal: to help perspective clients overcome or decrease the fear and apprehension of being an inpatient mental health client.

Objective: to help clients understand the dangers of masking mental health symptoms with drugs and alcohol. This can subsequently lead to a dual diagnosis, which makes treatment more complicated.

The information in this book is not meant to teach, instruct, prevent diagnoses, or treat mental health. This is the author's experience of thirty-one years as a mental health nurse.

Contents

Chapter 1   My Journey to Mental Health 1

Chapter 2   Mental Health Journey Continued..... 5

Chapter 3   Mental Health Journey Continued... 12

Chapter 4   Summary of The Baker Act Law 17

Chapter 5   Mental Health Home Care 24

Chapter 6   Community Mental Health 27

Chapter 7   Note to Parents 31

Chapter 8   My Specialty 34

Chapter 9   A Father's Plea 36

Chapter 10   Mental Health and Drug Abuse 40

Chapter 11   Managing Seniors' Mental Health ... 45

Chapter 12   Mental Health and Gun Violence 48

Chapter 13   Suicide and Mental Health 52

Chapter 14   Mental Health and Homelessness 56

Chapter 15 List of Some Medications

Used in Mental Health Treatment...60

Chapter 16 Discharge Planning..........................64

Chapter 17 Mental Health During a Pandemic...67

Chapter 18 Conclusion...74

Chapter 19 Non-Compliance With Medication....78

Introduction

Becoming a Nurse

I graduated as a registered nurse from Pace University in Pleasantville, New York in 1982. I immediately began my employment at a large teaching hospital in the Bronx, New York. At Montefiore Hospital, I was immediately placed on a medical surgical unit with the main focus on orthopedic surgeries. As I began my new career as a registered nurse, I was very excited and looking forward to learning as much as I could. My colleagues and head nurse shared with me that they were impressed with the way I communicated with my patients and with the staff. They thought I would do very well in mental health care. They mentioned that one of my patients had never been called by his name until I came. No one ever thought to buy a cake when it was someone's birthday until I came. My patient, Mr. S, began talking. I would start conversations with him because I cared for him. He would tell me about his family and his face would light up. He would say to me that I was working too hard. I would tell him how much I enjoyed taking care of my patients, watching them recover, and seeing them discharged. I told him that it was most rewarding when a patient was ill and then discharged home.

I was really enjoying my work on this unit. One Sunday, the supervisor called me and asked if I could come in to help with some emergency surgeries. I asked if there was a nurse in charge and she said yes. I left my husband and children that Sunday afternoon and went into work on my day off.

When I arrived, the unit seem chaotic. A patient was in the hallway waiting for a bed in ICU. The nurse in charge was floated to our unit, and she asked me if I would take charge since this was my unit. I agreed, although this meant coming in late, taking my assignment, and reading the report on all twenty-six patients on the unit. I also had to help nurses who needed help or had questions, and waiting to give report to the next shift.

After being there for two hours, I called the office of the supervisor, Mrs. Hines but she did not answer. Another hour passed without a call back, so I called the ICU attending physician. He was furious. Mrs. Hines called me after she received a call from the doctor and asked me, "Who do you think you are?"

I responded, "My name is Brenda Antoine. I currently am the nurse in charge of the second floor. Do you want me to stay or leave? I have a patient who has been waiting for an ICU bed all day."

She informed me that I had no business calling the doctor. I immediately realized the doctors must have some God complex. I personally never gave up my seat to a doctor when he or she arrived on the unit, like the other nurses did. I knew that day I would not be staying at Montefiore for any length of time.

I, however, kept running into trouble. One night, I was at work and one of my patients was very ill. Even though I was fairly new, I could recognize when one of my patients was in trouble I checked the patient's laboratory results and observed several abnormalities. I concluded that the patient could go into renal failure. I called the nursing office. As I was told during orientation, there is always someone there to help if you needed it.

The secretary laughed and said, "Who told you that?"

I said we all were told this while in orientation. I realized there was no help. Another nurse told me to put the lab results in the doctor's mailbox. I was very uncomfortable doing this, so I called my friend and mentor Hyacinth, a senior nurse. I told her the lab values. She reassured me that in the morning was all right for the doctor to receive it.

I knew I would not stay in medicine/surgery. That week, I applied to the Bronx Municipal Hospital Psychiatric Unit. Some of my colleagues had suggested that I would be a great psychiatric nurse. I left Montefiore Hospital.

Chapter 1: My Journey to Mental Health

I was hired at Bronx Municipal Hospital to work in the psychiatric unit in 9 East. The hospital had ten floors and the ninth and tenth floors were psychiatric units. I did two weeks of orientation, after which my shift was 7:00 a.m. to 3:30 p.m.

The first day I arrived on the unit, I was greeted by the head nurse, the doctors, and all other staff members. It was a very warm and accepting environment. Everyone would help me during the day. I carefully observed the unit routine, and before I knew it, I was taking change some days under supervision. I got good at it.

The assistant head nurse was switching units and I was asked to replace her. I was amazed because I had only been there for about four months.

The director of nursing called me before I had completed six months and informed me that Health and Hospital Corporation was supervising an internship for nurses in the corporate group. Two nurses from the hospital would participate in the internship. It would run for six months from 8:00 a.m. to 4:00 p.m. Monday to Friday. We would be paid. I and another nurse with whom I was in orientation would attend the class at Bellevue Hospital in Manhattan. The instructors were extremely knowledgeable and we learned a lot. After the six months, we returned to Bronx Municipal. When I returned to 9 East, I found that the program made working on the unit much easier. I was able to manage the unit, run community meetings, medication groups, staff meetings, and suicide assessment activity groups, deliver morning reports, and much more.

I remember being in school at Pace and being confused. The lectures in psychiatry never made sense. I remember asking my instructor Ms. Feldman for more help. She said, "Don't worry. You always get an A in everything else."

I said, "But I would like to get an A in psych."

She said, "Don't worry."

I got a C in her class. That was the only time I ever received a C in a nursing class. When she handed out the evaluation form, I wrote, "You could have made it easier by organizing the lectures this way."

Problem

signs and symptoms

nursing assessment

nursing implications

intervention

treatment or care

evaluation

organizing nursing lectures

In my opinion, this would have made it much easier to understand.

I was offered the assistant head nurse position. My duties changed slightly and involved more supervision. My head nurse said to me one day, "You are good at this job—very good. Maybe you want to look elsewhere to move up because I'm not leaving."

I responded by telling her that I enjoyed working with her and would like to learn more. She smiled. She was really very knowledgeable.

Chapter 2: Mental Health Journey Continued

By then, I realized that I was pregnant with my third child and had to take some time off.

One morning while in the hospital, the assistant director of nursing called me and said, "How are you? I would like to let you know that we have an administrative, head nurse position we would like to offer to you."

I responded, "I had my baby yesterday. I have not decided yet when to return to work."

She said, "Take your time. We will hold this position until you feel ready to return."

I had my baby on May 7 and returned to work on August 15 leaving my baby with a family member. My husband also took a night shift so he would be available if needed in the daytime.

I arrived on my new unit 9 West on August 15

I felt very welcomed. My director and assistant were also there to greet me. I mainly observed the first day.

As I continued in my first leadership role in mental health, I laid out my objectives. They are simple but very important in mental health safety. Every day, my plan was to manage my goals and objectives.

Goal: My daily goal was to prevent injury to all patients and staff.

Objective: to maintain a safe, therapeutic environment for all patients and staff.

My Daily Schedule

7:00 a.m.: Arrive on unit. Walk the unit and identify every patient, including the ones I believe would soon be in crisis by observing their behavior

7:45 a.m.: Morning report from the night shift

8:00 a.m.: Give an assignment to every nursing staff member. Patients who had made a suicide attempt or verbalized a suicide plan were assigned staff member. The staff member has to observe the patient no farther than arm's length. This staff member must be able to physically intervene with that patient immediately in an emergency or possible attempt. This is called 1:1 observation.

When the doctor has written an order to discontinue 1:1 observation, we then place the patient on a schedule to be checked every fifteen minutes; this is known as close observation. Here,

7

arm's length is not required. Once close observation is discontinued, all patients are checked every half hour for safety. This part of the assignment is one of the most important observations. It helps you keep the clients safe while they all are in your care. It also allows communication between staff and patients.

The nursing staff report to the doctors which clients were compliant with their medication and which were able to stay in control without becoming aggressive with staff, family members, or other clients. They also report which patients have been attending daily activity and unit participation groups. Most of all, nurses report those who are able to verbalize that they are no longer suicidal and indicate a place and person they could be discharged to.

It is every staff member's number one priority to help each patient maintain control. When a patient becomes so anxious that he or she loses control, becomes out of touch with reality, or becomes psychotic, it's all hands on deck.

We assign one person to speak while also getting down to eye level. It is important that the staff let the client know no one will hurt that person and that we were there to help him or her. Sometimes, we must administer emergency medication. If there is none ordered, we notify the doctor.

Other Diagnoses: Anxiety and Depression

Bipolar disorder is an affective disorder characterized by mood changes.

Schizophrenia is a thought disorder presenting with hallucinations, delusions, and withdrawal. I tell patients they have a problem with the way they think and speak when they ask.

Schizoaffective is schizophrenia compounded with an affective disorder, such as bipolar disorder.

Dual diagnosis means two disorders presenting

simultaneously, for example, depression with alcohol abuse.

One day, my director called me to her office five minutes after I arrived. A lady showed up at her office for a job interview. She said to me, "How are you?"

I responded, "How are you?"

She said, "What are you doing here?"

I said, "I work here."

My director said, "Since you two know each other, Brenda, why don't you do the interview." This lady was my instructor in psychiatry from Pace University.

We began the interview and, three questions in, I realized she would not fit well with my staff and even our clients. She still seemed disorganized in the way she answered questions. I told her she would hear from us. I told my director my reasons for not hiring her. She said she trusted my decision, so we did not hire her. Later on, I thought I should have used this opportunity as a teaching moment and as a model for how to treat staff and patients. We all interacted with, helped, and respected each other.

Chapter 3: Mental Health
Journey Continued

By then, I had completed four years on 9 West at Bronx Municipal Hospital. I decided to move to Florida because of affordable housing, the more temperate weather, and to leave a bad marriage behind.

I arrived in Florida and was able to join the psychiatric staff at Sand Lake Hospital as an assistant head nurse for inpatient mental health. I loved the job and the people I worked with. My job was to do all of the staff teaching. I found out that the newly enacted Baker Act was a challenge for all. The Baker Act was almost equivalent to a two-physician signature certificate that we used in New York. I obtained a Baker Act handbook and attended a Baker Act class.

I found out that the people teaching the class did not understand the Baker Act. The Baker

Act admissions were essentially divided between voluntary and involuntary admission. A patient who was admitted involuntarily was not allowed to go out on a pass. Being involuntarily admitted meant the patient was a danger to himself or herself or others. This unit did send involuntary patients out on day passes.

When I challenged the out-on-pass order, the staff would respond by saying, "That's because you came from New York." I was overreacting, they claimed.

They did it anyway. The following day was my day off. One of the nurses called me and asked if anyone on the unit had called me. I responded, "No." She told me the patient I warned them about sending out on pass was in the emergency room. He had taken an overdose while out on pass. Fortunately, he was unsuccessful.

When I returned to work the next day, no one could face me. Finally, I was approached by my head

13

nurse and a social worker. They admitted that I had a better understanding of the Baker Act and wanted me to teach the employees, including the doctors. I reminded them that the hospital was a Baker Act receiving facility, so we had to be prepared. That meant that all Baker Act clients had to be taken to the nearest Baker Act receiving facility.

I encountered another problem at this facility. It made me begin wondering if I chose the best facility.

A twenty-nine year-old white male stopped me on my way to my office, as patients often do when I arrive on the unit. I was shocked when this patient said to me that the night before, he felt suicidal. He got up in his room looking for something he could use to kill himself but was unable to find anything. He became frustrated and went back to bed. I asked him whether he was suicidal now. He said yes. When I asked how he would do it, he said he thought he could use his pants and his roommate's pants on the door. I immediately placed him on suicide precaution, which is 1:1 observation by a staff member within arm's length at all times.

I called the doctor and got no response, so I left a message with the secretary at his office at 9:15 a.m. I kept the patient on suicide precaution all day. We call it nursing 1:1 if we are unable to get the doctor's order at the time. I finally left work at 5:25 p.m. This doctor habitually arrived late, perhaps to avoid working with me. This staff member said that when they explained the situation to him, his response was not to let me see that patient first, but to ask, "Who does she think she is?" Apparently, his plan was to discharge the patient that day. However, I had put the patient on 1:1 observation. A discharge would seem like a violation to a reviewer. Who would discharge someone on the same day that person was on suicide watch?

I am very sorry, but I believe if a client's insurance

runs out, especially if the facility used up his days, I'm only interested in saving that person's life regardless of insurance status.

I was called in for questioning the next morning. I explained to the administration that should I experience any backlash for attempting to save someone's life, I would fight them in court and use the media to my advantage. I would be willing to go all the way to the Supreme Court. They called in another doctor to evaluate the patient. She had to stay on her colleague's (the doctor's) side, so her assessment was that she could not definitely say if he was suicidal or not. She was not sure.

My job, I believe, is always to be an advocate for my patient.

Needless to say, my patient remained on the unit until he verbalized that he was not suicidal anymore seven days later. I was also able to convince the insurance company to pay the additional seven days.

Chapter 4: Summary of The Baker Act Law

The Baker Act law was proposed by Congresswoman Maxine Baker of Florida in 1981, and it passed.

The purpose of the law was to protect the mentally ill. However, due to lack of knowledge and understanding of the law, many professionals and caregivers frequently use the law against the mental health patient. For example, I have heard so many approach a client and say, "If you don't stop, I will Baker Act you and you will be locked up for a long time." They could instead say, "I see that you need help. There is a law, especially for people who need help. It allows you to speak to a professional who can help you. Sometimes, you may have to go to the hospital where you will receive the most help, and work with people who will understand what you need."

In the United States, I am amazed that many more states don't use the Baker Act. I know in New York, there is a similar system called the 2PC, or the Two-Physician Signature or certificate. There are similarities between the two.

The Baker Act concentrates on two types of admissions. Voluntary admission is when a patient recognizes he or she needs help and requests admission. Sometimes, it's as easy as realizing that he or she has no medication.

The Baker Act encourages the voluntary admission of persons for psychiatric care, but only when they are able to understand the decision and its consequences and are able to exercise their rights for themselves. A client may be admitted voluntarily, but must be eighteen years old or older. A person seventeen years of age and under must have the admission signed by a guardian. NB. A minor can only be admitted on a voluntary if willing and upon application of his or her guardian. A hearing to verify the voluntariness of consent is held. A facility may not admit a person on a voluntary basis who has been adjudicated or incapacitated.

A person, relative, friend, or attorney may request a discharge on a voluntary admission either verbally or in writing. The client must be discharged within twenty-four hours, unless the doctor believes the person is a danger to himself or herself or others. In this case, he or she may initiate an involuntary admission.

Involuntary Admission: A person may be taken to a Baker Act facility involuntarily if the patient refuses voluntary admission.

Without care, the client may cause bodily harm to himself or herself or others.

The patient is likely to suffer from neglect as well. An involuntary admission has four parts.

(1) Involuntary: 3052a A law enforcement officer (LEO) can take a person into custody and have the person admitted under the Baker Act 52A law. This must be initiated by a law enforcement officer.

Involuntary 52B must be initiated by a physician, psychologist, mental health counselor (LMITC), licensed social worker (LCSW), practitioner, or registered nurse in a town of fifty thousand or fewer.

An ex parte order may be initiated by a family member, caretaker, or friend. A petition is made to the court indicating that this person is posing a danger to himself or herself and/or others. Failure to receive treatment will result in danger to the patient and others. Whichever type of admission a patient receives, we all must observe the following in regards to the patient's rights.

Each patient has the right to individual dignity and treatment, to express informed consent, and to receive quality treatment. Each patient has the right to communicate; he or she must be able to use the phone to report abuse. Each patient has the right to care and custody of his or her personal effects. The patient has the right to vote in public elections and to habeas corpus. The patient has the right to treatment and discharge planning, to select a representative, and to having his or her information remain confidential.

Violations of any rights or abuse of any privileges makes the violator liable for damages as determined by law.[1] N.B.

A Baker Act 3032 may be filed by the physician who initiates a first opinion and writes an order for

---

[1] Department of Mental Health Law and Policy, *2014 Baker Act: The Florida Mental Health Act User Reference Guide*, Tallahassee, FL: Department of Children and Families, Mental Health Program Office, 2014, pdf, https://www.myflfamilies.com/sites/default/files/2023-03/2014%20Baker%20Act%20Manual_0.pdf (accessed September 12, 2023).

a second opinion. The doctor who writes a second opinion must sign it within twenty-four hours, and it is then taken to be filed in the mental health court. This is usually because the doctors believe the patient needs a longer time to show improvement. The second opinion doctor usually goes to court. The client's guardian or family member is usually asked to attend. If the judge denies the doctor's request, then the patient has to be discharged. This usually occurs if a patient on a 52a or 52b refuses to sign a voluntary admission and receive help voluntarily.

Possible Changes to the Baker Act

From my experience, there are times when the seventy-two hours given to the physician to evaluate a patient are insufficient. When the seventy-two-hour period is nearing completion, the doctor may ask the client if he or she would sign a voluntary admission. This only happens after the doctor decides that the patient is now competent. If the patient refuses, this precedes a court hearing.

I find that patients do much better if we have about one week to care for them. This includes observing them for response to the medication regimen. The doctors should be trusted to medicate a client in an emergency because it is sometimes difficult to locate a patient health care proxy. This person must sign during an emergency to help a patient regain control.

Chapter 5: Mental Health Home Care

I saw an advertisement for a psychiatric home care nurse to make home visits.

I applied for the job and was hired at Columbia Home Care. I had no home care experience, but I knew mental health and medical surgical nursing, which is why I was hired. I did well visiting my mental health patient for a daily assignment and medication teaching on psychiatric drugs as needed. If the client also had a medical and/or surgical diagnosis, I was able to monitor all of it.

As I gained experience, I began to see eight or nine patients per day. I enjoyed my work, but my supervisor said that I was taking too long with the patients. I explained that while the company allowed one hour per visit, a psychiatric patient recently hospitalized would take much longer. She did not understand mental health. I explained that I am able to do an assessment and a dressing for a medical surgical patient in one hour. A psychiatric patient, however, requires time to establish trust. Then there must be time for an interview, for observing family dynamics, and checking their medication to verify medication compliance. I need at least ninety minutes.

Some psychiatric patients request that you have coffee with them when you come. For some reason, these patients are sensitive with fairly good insight and can usually tell if someone genuinely cares about them. I continued to work with my mental health clients the way I learned how. No one could change the way I worked with them because all I cared about was to do what was best for them.

I soon gained recognition. The supervisor told me that she admired the way I stood up for my patients. I eventually was promoted as they needed another supervisor.

My nursing style paid off. During a state inspection, I had to accompany a state inspector. The inspector was very impressed with the fact that when we visited patients, the patients knew me by name and would start a conversation with me. Needless to say, they did very well during the inspections. I teach young nurses how to do their jobs the right way every day and they will never have to worry.

This beautiful job soon came to an end when I took a two-week vacation. When I returned, I was told that the office had to be closed and I no longer had a job. Allegedly, our previous governor, who was one of the owners of our company, was accused of defrauding Medicare by upcoding diagnoses. This, to me, was an allegation that no one could prove. I had to find a job so I could take care of my three children. I quickly found employment at a nearby community mental health hospital.

Chapter 6: Community Mental Health

I was hired at Park Place Behavioral Health by a nurse who was once a member of my staff at another hospital. She actually told me she did not have a position but would like me to come on board to help her.

The unit was a crisis stabilization unit, and I was happy to join the team. I was back in familiar territory.

My director left soon after I was hired. When she left, I did my best to keep the facility in compliance with the state regulations. I felt somewhat uncomfortable since I was the last nurse hired. However, I was very aware of how to effectively manage a crisis stabilization unit, keep the facility in compliance, and teach the staff what they needed to know.

About two months later, the CEO approached me.

She said the director had told him before she left that I was the only nurse she felt could do her job. He offered me the job. No salary was negotiated, but I expected a raise for this management position. I had already done it for two months and been paid three dollars an hour after 5 p.m. for being on twenty-four-hour call. After we hired a new human resources director, he was amazed that my salary was so low. He did a comparative analysis in the area and brought me into the midrange of what others with my title and responsibilities were making.

About six months later, the CEO decided he could not pay me. He said, "You are a great worker. There is nothing wrong with your work, but we can't afford to pay you. We must lay you off."

They gave me $7000 and requested I sign a non-disclosure agreement. I signed it and left. I took the money and started my own business, but still explored my options. I started to recall events during my employment and this one stuck with me.

One morning, I came in and was told they had a hard night. A patient was secluded, and the staff on 1:1 sat at the door. I saw the patient asleep and asked the staff member to take him out of seclusion. He asked me if I was serious. I said yes and told him to check the observation board. The patient had been sleeping for the past four and a half hours. A nurse is supposed to initial the board every hour, but it was not done. I told both the nurse and the technician I wanted an incident report.

The client was in good control for almost five hours and still kept in seclusion. I sat with the patient and spoke to him. He told me he attended University of Florida and he came from Tennessee. call and save me the phone I asked his permission to contact his parents. They were sobbing when he told them he was in the hospital. He asked me to accompany him to see the doctor, and I was happy to do that. This incident stuck with me as I imagined my own son being away at school and alone.

I assisted his parents in finding accommodation in the area so they could visit their son. He was the middle child of three children. They thanked me for helping him. Their son was eventually discharged into their care. This is another example of how college could be stressful to young adults.

Chapter 7: Note to Parents

Dear Parents,

I am writing to you as another parent. As parents, we all dread experiencing one of our own kids succumbing to a mental health diagnosis. If you have a few kids, please remember that the one who requires the most intervention by you, who does not pay attention in school or complete assignments, or who is always testing limits, may need psychiatric testing. It may be a good idea to obtain a referral from your doctor for testing. Most testing costs about $400 unless you have insurance.

Please also pay attention to your young adult child between the ages of eighteen and twenty-six. This is usually the age they may be in college, and college is one of the most stressful events in a young person's life. If your kid is at risk for schizophrenia, this is usually the time when it will probably manifest.

If you have a teenager who begin using drugs or alcohol, this may be to mask symptoms they are experiencing. Most who end up with a mental health diagnosis have used substances to cover up symptoms of bipolar disorder, depression, or even schizophrenia.

Please don't assume that all your children must go to college. Some are more fragile than others and really cannot handle the stress of college. My son came to me and said, "Mom, can I move from University of Florida and go to Valencia, which is a two-year college, then go back to UCF later?" I said yes without asking why. I knew I raised him and he would make good decisions. He then explained that UCF holds classes in an auditorium with over one hundred students. Valencia classes were much smaller. I knew it would make him feel more comfortable. While at Valencia, he took the test for the US Air Force and passed. I reluctantly allowed him to go. He had a good career in the Air Force and he is now an IT instructor. I trusted his decisions.

I trusted him to make a sound decision and he completed college in the Air Force. Trust your kids. If they have an alternative to college, listen and work with them. You will be a happy parent.

Best wishes to you all,

Brenda

Chapter 8: My Specialty

Because mental health was my specialty and my passion, I could not stay away.

I applied at Lakeside Alternatives. They were in the planning stage of opening a medical unit on the fourth floor. I was hired to start working on opening up that new unit. Opening a new unit was a great experience. Several doctors I already knew started with me. The medical director was awesome. We would give him a list of families who called to speak to him and he returned every family's call. He also used the call to obtain his clients' histories. Like every other institution, many days I would have to go down to the central receiving center (CRC) because there was no one else in the building who could work both areas.

My doctor notified administration that whenever he was on the unit, he did not want me to be taken away because I facilitated the rounds and helped staff stay in compliance. With all that was expected of the staff, they described me as the glue that kept everything together and everyone in touch. At this hospital, we admitted a large amount of indigent patients. Everyone was treated well. This staff was always fully committed to the patients' well-being.

Lakeside Alternatives is a unique mental health system with two locations: one on the west side and one on the east side of Orlando. These include residential and daily clinics. When we assessed a client in CRC, we sometimes had to admit or transfer the client to the east side crisis unit. We were located on the west side of Orlando.

Chapter 9: A Father's Plea

As I walked down the hallway of my unit, a tall gentleman approached me in tears. He said, "Miss Brenda, please help me save my daughter."

I responded, "Who is your daughter sir?"

He stated, "CiCi." (This is name I used for confidentiality.)

I said I would do my best to get her the care she deserved, which is the best care.

He said, "I have heard about you." I brought him to my office and explained that we were dealing with a dual diagnosis. We found THC, cocaine, and ETOH in her system. Since the treatment team already decided that they would refer her to long-term care, I asked to evaluate her case again.

I requested that she be started on two protocols: the ETOH protocol and the cocaine protocol. We use the protocol suboxone Ativan. Once we completed the protocol, we started to work on the bipolar disorder. She stayed longer than most clients. Eventually she was able to be discharged for outpatient treatment. Her father thanked me. Most patients spend three to five days in this crisis unit. She had no insurance and spent thirty-seven days there after discharge.

I ran into CiCi at the grocery store. She looked well and happy. When she saw me, she wanted to pay for my groceries with her food stamps. I told her I could not accept anything from a patient. We are not even allowed to speak to the clients out in the community. I was so happy to see her. She looked well. She said, "I have to tell my dad I saw you." I was so happy that she was doing well.

It is immensely rewarding to run into your mental health clients in the community and see the ones who are doing well. On the other hand, you see the ones who are not. You are unable to immediately intervene. I have bought shoes and food when I see them barefooted in the neighborhood.

Christmas is usually difficult for me. I pick up presents and distribute them, mostly to the ones who are homeless. I buy McDonald's gift cards to make sure they have something to eat.

What I think would help them avoid the revolving door effect is to identify an organization to manage them. They can go every week and withdraw enough for the week from their checks. Kissimmee, Florida needs a shelter for the mentally ill. If I had the funds, I would build it. I was told by someone that a community pastor wanted to use a building of his, but the city of Kissimmee would not allow him to install the showers. There is no alternative, so homeless mentally ill clients walk the streets of Kissimmee, Florida.

Most mental health hospitals have an increase census at the end of the month Because clients' funds have run out, they come into the hospital and try to be discharged before check day. Some of them, maybe a group of about eight, for about $7.00 per person, rent a hotel room for the day so they could shower that day only. That's a smart and positive sign for this type of group. They shower and sleep in the hotel room for one night and the cycle starts over at the beginning of every month.

Chapter 10: Mental Health and Drug Abuse

Substance abuse is responsible for a large number of mental health admissions. Young adults may begin to experience hallucinations and delusions, which are signs and symptoms of both bipolar disorder and schizophrenia. Most people will attempt to mask symptoms with alcohol. Then, they try marijuana. When that doesn't help, they try crack or cocaine. Before they realize it, they have an addiction. It is that simple.

We must refrain from calling each other's children drug addicts. Can you imagine the trauma these young people experience when battling mental health symptoms? They become confused, not knowing what's happening to them.

They feel alone. Some seek out their primary physicians while trying to withdraw from the substances. They experience aches and pain. The doctor makes it worse by ordering them something for pain, which they also become dependent on.

Eventually, they check into the hospital. Instead of a diagnosis for bipolar disorder, for example, NOS they are also diagnosed with substance abuse disorder.

Some even go as far as heroin. If anyone believes it is easy to withdraw from heroin, it is not. Most end up returning to heroin to obtain relief from the withdrawal symptoms. They go back to using the drug.

Please don't label anyone's child as an addict. Instead, offer help to him or her because the person needs it. Even if the person rejects help, you must keep trying to help. I live in a town where I have worked as a registered nurse for two of the hospitals and as a mental health home care nurse. I sometimes try to hold tears back as I drive through my community.

If drugs are involved, we have to invoke the

Marchman Act in addition to the Baker Act once we have stabilized the mental disorder.

The Florida Marchman Act is a civil procedure that allows friends and family of substance abusers to confidentially petition the court to obtain an assessment order. This requires stabilization at a long-term treatment facility for up to five days. It also allows the judicial system to temporarily detain an individual involuntarily for emergency care of an addiction.

The CIWA scale is used for alcoholism assessments. We check a person's vital signs. The CIWA has a range of zero to seven, except for orientation, which has a range of zero to four. We check for nausea and vomiting, tremors, paroxysmal sweats, anxiety, agitation, visual disturbance, headache, orientation, and clouding of sensorium. A score of zero to seven (except for orientation) means the patient must be assessed every four hours. If all scores are below eight for seventy-two hours, then you may discontinue use of CIWA assessment.

Many doctors use Ativan. Other substances may be sedatives, hypnotics, nicotine, cannabis, cocaine, amphetamines, opiates, morphine, heroin, or meperidine. *Substances* refers to agents taken automatically to alter mood or behavior.

The opioid crisis requires a mandate like the Marchman Act. Treatment is free of charge with absolutely no cost to the client. More state hospitals should provide substance abuse treatment.

Nurses are required to submit to opioid training CEUs every two years. I believe police officers and teachers should also be required to fulfill these CEU requirements.

Some Clinical Signs of Substance Abuse

Alcohol: Appearance of unsteady gait. Levels peak by the second day.

Sedative: Unsteady gait

Nicotine: Nausea, vomiting, loss of appetite.

Cannabis: Red eyes, tachycardia (rapid pulse), dry mouth, euphoria.

Cocaine: Red eyes, pacing, euphoria, talkativeness, hypervigilance, hallucinations.

Amphetamines: Pupil dilation, sweating or chills, high or low blood pressure, impaired judgment, impaired social functioning, agitation.

Opiates: Pinpoint-size pupils, decreased blood pressure and pulse, slurred speech, impaired judgment.

Chapter 11: Managing Seniors' Mental Health

Unfortunately, seniors really do not belong on an acute mental health unit.

When a senior arrives in a mental health facility, he or she is usually in one of the stages of dementia, early Alzheimer's, or withdrawal from Xanax. If the person is coming from home, alcohol is usually in the mix. The mini cog is usually used for assessing the elderly. This consists of a three-item recall and a drawing of a clock.

During the assessment of a senior, we frequently find that the person is withdrawing from Xanax, which many practitioners order for these patients. We personally believe it is not a good idea because they withdraw when they are out of the medication. This causes severe behavior changes. Many seniors are sent from the nursing home to an acute psychiatric unit.

Seniors should not be Baker Acted. Nursing homes should have a few psychiatrists on their medical staff. The medical doctor usually sees the patients once each month. NB Any client with a diagnosis of mental retardation also should not be Baker Acted. Seniors in any of the four stages of dementia should not be Baker Acted. The nursing home sends them to psychiatry if they cannot sleep, if they are sundowning, yelling, and/or disruptive. Most psychiatric facilities prefer to care for seniors on a special psychiatric unit[2] with a practitioner on staff.

When seniors live alone at home, they also tend to be non-compliant with their medication. Sometimes this is due to memory deficit. Other times, they are just unable to manage. Families are sometimes instructed to use a pill organizer to improve and maintain compliance.

---

[2]

A full assessment is completed an all seniors during the course of the medication assessment. The assessor can usually obtain information about cognitive functioning. We also use the MO stick. Sometimes, a urinary tract infection can cause seniors' behavior to change as well. Checking their blood sugar is also important because abnormal blood sugar levels can cause behavior changes in some seniors. Whatever the assessment reveals, our goal is usually to get them back to familiar surroundings.

Chapter 12: Mental Health and Gun Violence

Mental health has played a big role in gun violence. The shootings that have stayed on my mind are Sandy Hook Elementary School, Columbine High School, Parkland High School, the Orlando nightclub, and Mother Emanuel Church. I frequently ask myself if I have the coping skills necessary to deal with losing one of my three children. The answer is no.

I admire the congresswoman whose goal is to make changes in gun violence laws. She is patiently waiting. She lost her son because he was playing loud music. I'm hoping someone helps her. I watched the president, with his gaming behavior, talking to the Parkland High School kids. He could not relate to what they just went through. All he could think about was his reelection and to avoid working against one of his largest donors, the NRA, which has basically been an obstacle.

What most people don't realize is that a large percentage of persons who purchase or own firearms have some type of mental illness. We can avoid such violence by putting a screening tool in place. I am a nurse and I need a background check to start a small business. Anyone who needs to purchase a firearm should be required to have a background check. This can be kept in a clearing house. Permit renewal should be required every five years. Attached please find a gun pre gun purchase evaluation.

Pre Gun Sale Evaluation

NAME:_____ AGE:_____ DOB: _____

must be age 21 or older

SSN	Yes	No
Hx of mental illness?	☐	☐
Currently on medication?	☐	☐

List of medications:	
Type of Firearm:	
Reason for Firearm:	

Have you ever been Baker Acted?	☐	☐
If yes, when?	Date:	
Ever been convicted of a crime?	☐	☐
Do you currently own a gun?	☐	☐
Do you drink alcohol?	☐	☐
If yes, how often?		

References:

1.		2.		3.	
Ph.		Ph.		Ph.	

Approve: Sig:		Disapprove Sig:	

Have you ever been convicted of a crime?	☐	☐

Please explain why a firearm is important to you.	

Is there anyone that you believe wants to hurt you or you would like to hurt?	☐	☐
Name and phone number of person		
Has the seller identified any red flags?	☐	☐

If yes, what are their comments?

_____

_____

_____

Chapter 13: Suicide and Mental Health

Suicidal ideation or suicide attempts are the most dreaded admissions to mental health facilities. You wonder what systems you must put in place while the person is in hospital. You also wonder how to implement and maintain a necessary network when the patient is discharged. Do you place the patient on suicide watch or one-to-one observation if the patient is still suicidal and has a plan? If the patient is suicidal but has no plan, the doctor may consider an antidepressant, then place the person on close observation (to be checked every fifteen minutes).

If the patient is suicidal or homicidal and a firearm is part of the plan, then we have a duty to warn others. One way to do this is through the police, who would go to the patient's residence and remove the firearm.

Antidepressants are frequently used. I also realize

that drug and alcohol are frequently involved in my assessment using the Uno sticks. The concerning thing to me is that suicide affected a cross section of diagnoses There is no one way to know who is likely to commit suicide. A depressed patient may have a history of being suicidal. Someone with bipolar disorder may have a history with suicidal ideation. and seem to be the most common diagnosis that make attempts on suicide and succeed in suicide The schizophrenic patient also may have a history of suicidal ideation.

My plan for reducing suicide is always to treat everyone as a suspect. As with any commensurable disease, substance abusers may have experienced a loss and become suicidal. This could be the loss of a loved one, especially a child, or the loss of a job, money, home, control, independence, a limb, a relationship, or many others. We need to be aware that people around us are quite likely to be suicidal.

Doctors treat the underlying diagnosis, which at times is suicidal thoughts and frequency.

Some doctors would actually try electroconvulsive therapy for chronic suicide attempts. This therapy may result in forgetfulness or memory loss. The hope is that the patient would not recall that he or she was once suicidal.

Adolescents have a significantly high incidence, but I believe the causes are different. They respond to pressure from mostly bullying during use and unhealthy relationships.

Seniors also commit suicide because of isolation and loss of independence. It is believed that when a person is depressed and has low energy, the chance of a suicide attempt is lower. However, once the person begins to come out of the depression and has more energy, the chance of a suicide attempt is more likely. a bipolar D/O perhaps the reason the bipolar leading in incidents when they are in a manic episode.

People without a mental health diagnosis can also become suicidal and/or homicidal. This is very disheartening. When an elderly person becomes suicidal and involves the spouse, it is a suicide and a homicide.

Chapter 14: Mental Health and Homelessness

Homelessness is the undiagnosed American disease. I live in Florida, but there is homelessness everywhere. In every state I have visited, there is homelessness. George Carlin once said, "We should use every golf course to ease homelessness." I agree. Let's start with Donald Trump in New Properties Jersey, or start in Miami and move north.

It has dawned on me recently that maybe I could file taxes for all the money I give to the homeless. I give money during bad weather. I give money for food frequently. I wonder if they could receive food stamps to purchase cooked food. They are grocery stores, the clothing stores, matter of fact they are everywhere There is such a fine line between homelessness and having a home. Shame on America.

I am a disabled single woman caring for veterans. I buy clothing, shoes, and food. I check on medications. I was informed by one of them that a pastor attempted to convert one of the buildings on his property. However, the city would not allow him to install showers. We must do our part to assist our fellow Americans who experience various misfortunes fighting to protect us and up end up homeless.

I spend about $80.00 per month, at least. This is such a small amount. If we all contribute $80.00 per month, think about the impact we can have on their lives and the satisfaction we would also receive. Can you believe that this large sector of the population would not be counted in the census 2020? What will happen to them? Many are veterans with PTSD. Did they fight to protect us so they can return home and live on the street?

They are frequently admitted to mental health facilities after being Baker Acted by the police. Most of them are aware of the criteria for admission, so they use it. You have to be a danger to yourself or others. Once admitted, they can have showers and three meals a day for a short period of seventy-two hours. This is no way to live, especially after you have served your country. This also at times holds a bed that could be otherwise assigned to someone really in crisis so that person does not have to end up in a medical bed in the hospital. It is such a ripple effect.

I met a young man recently who told me someone told him to come to Florida and he would get work. He came from Georgia. He showed me the back of the warehouse where he sleeps. He lights up as you hand him three dollars to buy something to eat. He stands next to a garbage can, using it as a table while he eats what is probably the only thing he would eat that day.

As the mother of a son who went into the service, the tears rolled down my cheeks. I walked away toward my car. He said, "Mamie man, don't forget to put on your seat belt, and put on your glasses which you took off to dry your tears." You could not address mental health without considering the homeless population.

Chapter 15: List of Some Medications Used in Mental Health Treatment

Frequently used medications are anti-psychotic/ neuroleptics used to decrease symptoms of psychosis such as delusions, hallucinations, and agitation. These include

- Haldol;

- Geodon;

- Risperdal; and

- Olanzapine.

Neuroleptics do have side effects, such as EPS, NMS, neuroleptic malignancy syndrome, tardive dyskinesia, dry mouth, and dystonia. Side effects can include ocular gynicmotion (the eyes roll up as if the person is looking at the ceiling) and tongue protrusion.

For akethesia, patients can be given medication for

Parkinson's disease, such as benztropine. Benadryl can relieve the side effects. anti-depression to teach depression i.e.

Antidepressants, including Prozac and citalopram, are used to improve mood.

Mood stabilizers, like Seroquel, can be used to treat bipolar disorder.

For anxiety, Buspar or Lorazepam are often prescribed.

Attending the nursing staff: medication group is a daily responsibility. It may be conducted as follows.

Nurse: This is our daily medication group from Monday to Friday. The purpose of this group is to allow all of you to ask questions and receive feedback about your medication. Please raise your hand and wait until I call on you.

Patient: Is the medication really good for me? I stopped taking the medication for two months and I felt fine until today.

Nurse: You should take your medication every day. The reason you felt OK for a while is because the body ist??? Medication, When medication is needed, the body releases medication that had built up. At some point, the medication that was stored becomes depleted. Therefore, you would start to decompensate and show symptoms, hence your reason for returning to the hospital for noncompliance with the medication drop box. This is a frequent reason for patient readmission.

Patient: What if I have an adverse reaction? Nurse: The doctor always *adds* medication that would prevent adverse effects when you are discharged. Usually, this would be Benztropine, Benadryl, Artane, or amantadine. When discharged, please order your medication when you have only three days left. Avoid direct sunlight. If you have dry mouth, you may want to keep some sugar-free hard candy with you. Your discharge planner will make sure you have information on your medication.

Chapter 16: Discharge Planning

Over the years, social workers have carved out their own department in mental health care. It is very important to have a thoughtful discharge plan and sh??? I have include the patient and their family mental??? what health has the highest reciv about prism rate yesterday pla??? Mental some describe it as the new??? The cause is usually 83/87 poor discharge planning start they will tell and now compliant with medication regime you it starts at admission a new mission all. If you ask a health care provider when does discharge planning start, he or she will tell you it starts at admission. 8 talk with family on admission all patients are assigned session is usually required before they show also to

A case manager, who is either a social worker or a nurse, will begin gathering information on the first day to facilitate a smooth and appropriate discharge arrangement. When the patient becomes more stable, we also require that the patient attend a discharge planning group. There, we provide instructions again on the importance of adherence to medication, instruct unbalancing rest with excuse the importance of proper diet, and avoiding the use of alcohol with medications. We stress the importance of attending to their personal hygiene, frequent showering, proper grooming, and proper clothing selection. Follow-up appointments are made. We must be careful to link the patient with the health care provider he or she seems most compatible with or who is very experienced with the particular diagnosis and or issues.

Lastly, we determine if the client is employed. social service usually provide them with a sick note to cover the lost time off children also receive a note. If an ISM client returns to the hospital in less than a month, we evaluate his or her medical records and discharge plan to see where we went wrong. We also encourage clients that though they met other patients and formed friendships, this is usually not a good idea. The reason is that all of them have problems they are addressing. Forming new relationships may take away from caring for themselves because people work on relationships. Friendships may be fine while the person is in the hospital under supervision, but they could become too complicated on the outside. Dealing with someone who has problems similar to the person's may be difficult.

Many patients also returned because they cannot afford the medication. Even with insurance, medications can be very expensive. As nurses, we obtain information for the doctors about choosing the discharge medication that is affordable. Teaching about medication side effects is another important part of the discharge plan. We instruct all clients on how to handle side effects from using hard? For y mouth calling 911 for emergency treatment, to like EPS.

Chapter 17: Mental Health During a Pandemic

As I complete my mental health journey, I cannot help but notice the amount of anxiety around me coming from friends and family. Of course, the reason for the increased anxiety is because we are in the middle of a pandemic. Because I am in the medical field, all of my friends and family gravitate toward me. I began organizing to try to keep us all safe. I mailed gloves and masks to the most vulnerable. The ones who needed some financial help I knew would ask, and they did. Now I realize I was at a point of experiencing a mental health crisis during the pandemic.

Because of my own comorbidities, I called the assisted living facility where I serve as the administrator. I decided to work from home. I was immediately able to update all the clients' treatment plans, immediately suspend visitations, and notify all next of kin. I also held a meeting with staff and provided instructions. They had to wear masks, wash their hands frequently, and practice social distancing. Anyone with comorbidities had the opportunity to work in an area with no physical contact, such as the office, kitchen, or laundry.

The patients also had to be instructed on the importance of wearing a face covering, frequent hand washing, and social distancing. Their treatment plans were updated.

Problem: Patient is at risk of infection related to COVID-19.

Intervention:

(1) Monitor temperature twice daily; if elevated, isolate and notify doctor.

(2) Instruct on frequent hand washing and importance of social distancing.

Staff Signature

B. Thigpen, RN

Lucky for me, I was in possession of PPE. As soon as I heard the virus was being spread by droplet infection, I did not wait for the CDC to recommend wearing a mask. They did it too late. My family and friends were wearing masks way before the CDC's announcement. I suggested it to my gym administrators, but I was ignored. I did not go to my gym from March 1.

I worked closely with the doctors. as many of our clients required sedatives, at times to stay calm. As they heard more information about COVID-19, they became more anxious. The staff was instructed to pay attention to the clients who already had a mental health diagnosis.

An added responsibility I took on was to check on my friends who decided to go in to work. At the end of the day, they would be physically and mentally drained. I encouraged them to call me no matter what time if they needed to talk. Some talked, some cried, and some just got downright mad at themselves.

As a nursing administrator, I frequently wrote the infection control policy and procedure, which every hospital unit must have. I felt blessed that I was in a position to help friends and families, although I was not physically going into the hospital. It is amazing how just wearing a mask, washing your hands, socially distancing, eating a balanced diet, and exercising can help a person stay healthy.

Finally, I, the patients, and the staff were tested biweekly. We have had all negative results. I believe everyone has learnt from this pandemic. Just the word *pandemic* is anxiety provoking. Can you imagine how it must make a person with a mental health diagnosis feel?

We all have a responsibility to reach out to each other.

Remind others that you are there for them and that they can call any time.

Ask how they feel. Reassure them that you will always be there for them.

Remind them to wear masks when out of the house.

Tell them they can call you if they feel sick. Remind them to practice social distancing.

All should invest in a thermometer.

Remind them to eat and stay hydrated.

Exchange movies, books, or games and talk about them.

Currently, there have been 200,000 COVID-related deaths. The president continues to hold rallies, with no social distancing and no one wearing a mask. I instruct my patients to avoid political discussions, so maybe I should take my own advice and just hope for a vaccine soon.

One of my daughters lost her best friend and her best friend's son. I hate to close with sadness. They both had comorbidities, so please be safe and follow CDC guidelines.

As a mental health nurse, I am concerned about the clients who live alone, the ones who experience feeling ill and die alone at home from COVID-19. There are the ones who become isolated and depressed, the ones who succumb to alcohol and other substances, and the ones who make it to the hospital but still have to die alone. I believe grieving starts at the point when you walk away from the hospital after you held your loved one's hand and watched him or her take that last breath.

But as Dr. Kübler-Ross pointed out, the stages of grief are denial, anger, bargaining, depression, and acceptance. How many families had the opportunity to go through all stages with a hope of a complete grieving process, which finally facilitated acceptance with the ability to move on?

Chapter 18: Conclusion

In conclusion these are my suggestions.

1. The Baker Act should be adopted in all fifty states

2. The Marchman act should be considered because it would save lives, especially with our current opioid crisis.

3. There should be a clearing house for the background checks of anyone applying for a firearm permit.

4. There needs to be oversight of drug companies. All mental health prescriptions should have capped prices. Remember, these clients are unable to work for the most part of their lives. How would they afford medications?

5. All states must receive funds to alleviate or eliminate homelessness.

6. A special task force must be set up in cities too. Homelessness is not even in those s***hole countries that the president mentioned. Have I seen homelessness of the magnitude I have in the US?

7. The State Department should be in charge of assisted living facilities. Nursing homes should provide more teaching to staff instead of their current punitive policy with? And closures they should teach and reteach staff utilization review

8. There needs to be more oversight of insurance companies. They say they are covering mental health care. However, a day after a patient makes a suicide attempt, they tell you to discharge the patient because they won't approve any more days in the hospital. When a client starts a new medication, he or she should automatically remain under

observation in the hospital for at least five to seven days.

9. We must fund schools so they can employ mental health staff, at least psychologists, licensed clinical social workers, or mental health nurses. Money for psychological testing by the beginning of junior high will help reduce gun violence.

10. Registered nurses' licenses need to be statewide. One state license should allow you to work in all fifty states. During pandemics, hurricanes, tornadoes, earthquakes, and other disasters, we need nurses to work in any state where they are needed without having to apply for a license in another state.

11. Health care workers and teachers should be able to go to college for free. After being a nurse for fifteen years, you should be able to take one class and become grandfathered

into a nurse practitioner role. This will ease the cost of medical care. The practitioner can work under the supervision of a doctor. This will also build trust efficiency of client as an outpatient an inpatient, can reduce the cost of medical care also.

Chapter 19: Non-Compliance With Medication

At any time on an inpatient medication unit, about 60 percent of the census is usually as a result of non-compliance with previously ordered medication. Sometimes, after obtaining past history, you realize that they stopped taking medications as far back as high school. Antidepressants may have been ordered. After a short time, parents saw an improvement and stopped the medications.

One of the main reasons for non-compliance is the cost of medications. In President Biden's latest healthcare and pharmaceutical review, he capped insulin at $35.00 per month. I wish, and I plan to request, that we do the same for anti-psychotics, neuroleptics, antidepressants, mood stabilizers, and other frequently used medications in mental health care. If we can start by controlling prices, we may definitely see a reduction in cases and, subsequently, in homelessness.

I believe many clients who are mentally ill and lack proper treatment eventually become homeless. Those who receive disability usually check into the hospital when they run out of money for food and medication.

Another reason for non-compliance, I believe, is insurance companies' inability to work closely with the patients and their healthcare providers. I have spent many hours trying to convince them that when we have a non-compliant patient who takes oral medication, we can begin an intramuscular dose that costs more upfront but lasts for two to three months at a time. This prevents the family from having to worry every day if the patient took his or her medication. An injection once every two to three months is better for the patient.

The third reason for non-compliance is the fact

that anti-psychotic medications have side effects that are very frightening to the patients. With EPS (extra pyramidal side effects), the patient may show dystonia (body stiffness), tongue protrusion, or ataxia, a nervous condition that affects coordination, balance, and speech. The doctor needs to add an anticholinergic like Cogentin, Benztropine, or amantadine. Even Benadryl helps. None of these should be taken without a doctor's order.

During a patient's hospital stay, I would usually convene a twice-weekly medication group. One of the most frequent questions patients ask is, "Ms. Brenda, how come I have not taken my medication for three months and I am OK?"

My response is usually, "Do you think you are OK? You are here in the hospital."

Then they will respond, "I guess I am not OK."

I would then state that it is never a good idea to stop taking your medication unless the doctor tells you to. However, the liver is your largest organ. One of the things the liver does is store some medication when you take it. At times when you stop taking your medication, the liver releases some as the body needs it. After a while, all that the liver stored is depleted. If you are not taking your medication when all is depleted, you now begin to decompensate and start showing signs and symptoms, and you will keep coming back to the hospital. Some people describe this process as the revolving door syndrome.

Bibliography

Department of Mental Health Law and Policy. *2014 Baker Act: The Florida Mental Health Act User Reference Guide.* Tallahassee, FL: Department of Children and Families, Mental Health Program Office, 2014. Pdf. https://www.myflfamilies.com/sites/default/files/2023-03/2014%20Baker%20Act%20Manual_0.pdf (accessed September 12, 2023).

Jarvis, Carolyn. *Physical Examination and Health Assessment.* 7th ed. Philadelphia, PA: Saunders, 2015.

Supporting Information Obtained from

(1) The Baker Act guide hand book by the state of Florida 2006, Department of children and families mental health program

(2) Jarvis Carolyn PhD APN CNP Seventh Edition

(3) Nursing handbook guide, Nursing 2016 The American Webster handy college dictionary, third edition

Google Information

Index

Anesthesia

Anxiety

Behavior

Bipolar

Compliant

Crisis

Decompensate

Depression

Dementia

Diagnosis

Dystonia

Escalate

Homicidal

Involuntary

Isolate

Miler

Paroxysmal

Prognosis

Recidivism

Revolving door

Schizophrenia

Senior

Voluntary

(4)

Thank You

I would like to thank my friend and mentor Hyacinth Martin for always being there for me, for encouraging me, and believing I am smart and I am a good nurse. Thanks to my cousins Bernadette Ifill and Marlene Young for believing that I am a working hand. Thanks for doing my chores when I would go to the library all day Saturday. Thanks to my late cousin Deborah Frederick. Thanks to my children, Dwayne, La Verne, and Shena Antoine, of whom I am proud for all their help. Thanks to my friends, to name a few, Marita Mason RN, Lynella Casting MSW, Faye Phillips, Gillian Clapham T'dcd, Patricia Dixon T'dcd, and Tamaja Travis for always believing in me and giving their support.

Taraya Travis, thank you.

About the Author

My Story

My name is Brenda Thigpen. I was born Brenda Haywood. I was married and have three children. I am currently a widow. I was born in Trinidad, West Indies, sometimes called the eighth wonder of the world for its pitch lake, one of our main sources of exports. I graduated from Southeast Port of Spain Secondary High School.

I migrated to Birmingham, England, where I became a state enrolled nurse. I was later admitted to West Bromwich Hospital to pursue my state-registered nurse certificate. I came to the United States and became a US citizen. I attended Pace University in Pleasantville, New York where I graduated as a registered nurse in 1982. I matriculated into the BSN program. Not long after my graduation, my career began to escalate successfully.

Soon, jealously was evident in my marriage and I noticed that I was becoming a battered wife. Domestic violence had reared its ugly head in an eighteen-year-old marriage with no warning. I was aware of what could happen to my children if I stayed, so I immediately begin making arrangements to leave.

After the first court hearing, where I felt that the courts were not providing me with the protection I needed, I came to Florida one weekend and bought a house. Later, I left in the middle of the night while my husband the abuser was at work I arranged my move for midnight. I took all I wanted and sent it ahead of me. I slept in a hotel near the airport and flew to Florida the following morning. I knew I would have to move to another state to feel safe.

Young women, or whoever is experiencing domestic violence, find a way to have a personal account. Save money. Don't stay; he will eventually kill you. Confide in someone. I taught a group at work on domestic violence, so all I had to do was put my own advice to work for me.

I continued my nursing career in Florida. I was able to care for my children as a middle-class worker, even though it meant working sixteen-hour shifts at times. I was able to pay for babysitting and still live fairly comfortably.

Don't be afraid of being alone. Take a chance on your life. I eventually remarried to a wonderful man who adopted my kids. He died after three years.

We are now Floridians even though they were born in New York. We are enjoying Florida weather.

As you see, mental health comes full circle. Please note that the first time an abuser hurts you is when you start to make arrangements to leave. You can call the domestic violence hotline. In some states, including Florida, you must do Domestic Violence

CEUs biannually for license renewal for nurses. I believe police officers and teachers should also be required to complete these biannual CEUs on domestic violence.

I was very fortunate to have been able to attend nursing school in the United Kingdom and the United States. This gave me the ability to excel in practical application and theory. God bless the UK and the USA.

COVID Response Chapter 18

1

As COVID-19 became a pandemic and a lockdown was initiated, I immediately became concerned for the college-age kids aged eighteen to twenty-six. My reason was that these kids are already stressed with school.

Imagine being secured in your parents' home. When you turn eighteen, you must leave, go to some archaic college dorm, and share a room with a complete stranger. You begin using alcohol to help reduce your anxiety, Then the alcohol loses its effectiveness. You take a pill from someone. When the pill stops working, you decide to try some white powder that you now put in your nose, or maybe something in a syringe. You now have to come to our emergency room, and we the medical team have to decide whether we should treat the drug use or the underlying mental illness.

Keep in mind that this is the age that mental illness, if you are predisposed, will begin to manifest itself. If people in this age group are not treated appropriately, they may manage to graduate only to join another vulnerable group: the twenty-six to forty-five year-olds. There was a time when the CDC identified this group as having the highest suicide lethality.

Parents, you may want to consider having your middle school and high school children tested. Add a psychiatric evaluation to their school physical so problems can be identified. Any predisposition to schizophrenia, bipolar disorder, depression, or anxiety can be treated early enough to assure a smoother transition from high school to college.

It would seem to me that in the freshman and sophomore years, it would be a good idea to initiate and maintain support groups. Give the students an opportunity to talk about college life and identify any problems or concerns they may have. A faculty member should be present so that parents can be notified of possible changes in their kids' behavior.

Early evaluation and treatment is most beneficial. I believe participation in the support group may help to deter some of the drug experimenting. A psychologist I worked with once told me I was naive if I believed that none of my children experimented with drugs. I later admitted to myself that if any of them did, it would have to be during their transition to college. I stopped tormenting myself, and approached the three of them individually. My youngest admitted to trying marijuana while the two older ones denied that they had.

As I reflect on that period of their lives, I could recall the time she withdrew, avoided much contact, and seemed impatient frequently. She lost a little weight, kept borrowing money from her siblings, and changed her attire from being meticulous to sloppy. She told me I kept commenting on her behavior, but the day I took her bedroom door off the hinges, I really scared her. I scared her enough, and told her I was ready to intervene.

She asked me not to tell anyone. I told her this was an all-hands-on-deck problem; the whole family would have to be involved. She promised it would stop. I said I would stop when she stopped.

Over the next three months, I did random dipstix, sometimes at 2:00 a.m. It was an experience.

Don't be afraid to confront. I learned from some evangelist on television that confrontation is an attempt to preserve a relationship. Don't be afraid speak to their friends and go into their rooms. Don't allow them to restrict you from any part of the house because you pay the rent or mortgage for the whole house. Insist on having dinner time and family time.

Keep confronting, or you will be defeated by drugs, alcohol, or mental illness. If the twenty-six to forty-five year-olds are not treated, they will have trouble keeping jobs and forming meaningful relationships. Good luck.

Brenda Antoine Thigpen, RN

NY Lic. #352389 FL Lic.
#1910182 GA Lic pending

1608 Regal Cove Ct., Kissimmee, FL 34744
Ph. 407-618-9195 Fax. 407-350-3713

Experience

2010–Present: Administrator, Neptune Manor ALF

2008–2010: Charge Nurse, New Facility 49 Acute beds Orlando, FL, Central Florida Behavioral Hospital, Mental Health

2007–2009: Nursing Director, Educare Legal Nurse Consulting Firm, Kissimmee, FL

2007–2008: Charge Nurse/Assistant to Court Liaison, Lakeside Behavioral Health Mental Health, Orlando, FL

2000–2007: Assistant Director of Nursing, Park Place Behavioral Health Care Crisis Stabilization, adult and children Mental Health, Kissimmee, FL

1998–2000: Clinical Supervisor and Case Manager, Columbia Home Care (Psychiatric and Medical Surgical Client Care), Kissimmee, FL

1995–1998: Case Manager, Visiting Nurse Association (VNA) Home Care, St. Cloud, FL

1990–1992: Staff Nurse/Evening Supervisor, Osceola Health Care Nursing Home, Kissimmee, FL

1988–1990: Assistant Nurse Manager, Orlando Regional Medical at Sand Lake Hospital (Inpatient Mental Health), Orlando, FL

1984–1988: Administrative Head Nurse, Health and Hospital Corporation at Jacobi Hospital (Inpatient Mental Health), Bronx, NY

1982–1984: Staff Nurse, Montefiore Hospital and Medical Center (Medical Surgical Nursing Affiliate of Albert Einstein Medical Center), Bronx, NY

1977–1982: Nursing Supervisor, East Haven Nursing Home LPN to RN, Bronx, NY

Education/Training

Pace University, New York

RN: Matriculated into BSN Program

ANA

Certification in Mental Health

Health and Hospital Corporation

Psychiatric Internship

American Red Cross

Health and Safety CPR and HIV instructor

Vickie Milazzo Institute

Certified Legal Nurse Consultant (CLNC)

Knowledgeable in Baker Act Laws and Florida Statues in Mental Health

Other Details

Utilization Review Manager

State of Florida Notary

ALF Consultant Instructor

www.ingramcontent.com/pod-product-compliance
Lightning Source LLC
Chambersburg PA
CBHW031122180526
45160CB00005B/52/J